YOUR KNOWLEDGE HAS VALUE

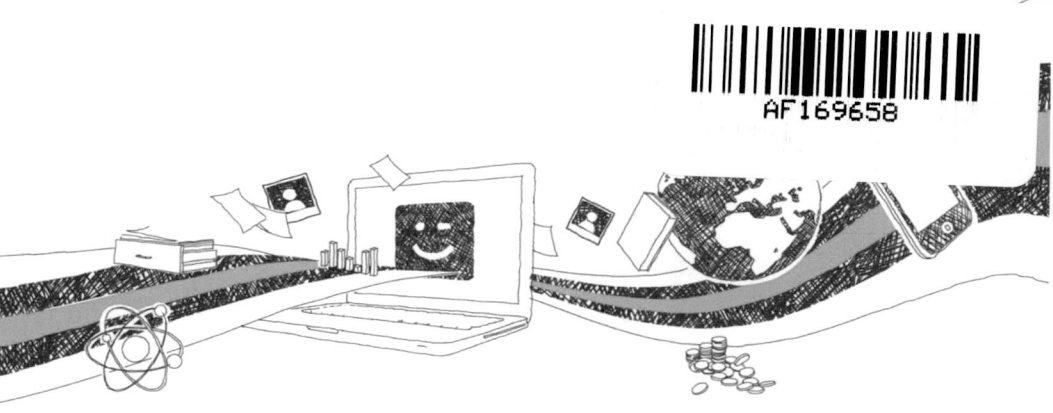

- We will publish your bachelor's and master's thesis, essays and papers

- Your own eBook and book - sold worldwide in all relevant shops

- Earn money with each sale

Upload your text at www.GRIN.com
and publish for free

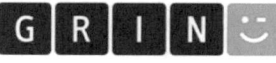

Bibliographic information published by the German National Library:

The German National Library lists this publication in the National Bibliography; detailed bibliographic data are available on the Internet at http://dnb.dnb.de .

This book is copyright material and must not be copied, reproduced, transferred, distributed, leased, licensed or publicly performed or used in any way except as specifically permitted in writing by the publishers, as allowed under the terms and conditions under which it was purchased or as strictly permitted by applicable copyright law. Any unauthorized distribution or use of this text may be a direct infringement of the author s and publisher s rights and those responsible may be liable in law accordingly.

Imprint:

Copyright © 2016 GRIN Verlag
Print and binding: Books on Demand GmbH, Norderstedt Germany
ISBN: 9783668646629

This book at GRIN:

https://www.grin.com/document/386039

Anonym

Organ donation. Does a decision for a donation make sense?

GRIN Verlag

GRIN - Your knowledge has value

Since its foundation in 1998, GRIN has specialized in publishing academic texts by students, college teachers and other academics as e-book and printed book. The website www.grin.com is an ideal platform for presenting term papers, final papers, scientific essays, dissertations and specialist books.

Visit us on the internet:

http://www.grin.com/

http://www.facebook.com/grincom

http://www.twitter.com/grin_com

GFS in 2016/2017
School subject: English

2016/17

Organ donation

Does a decision for a donation make sense?

Structure

1. In General – What is organ donation?.. 2
    The living donation

2. Process of organ donation – a race against death... 3

3. The situation of organ donations in Germany... 4
    The waitlist in Germany

4. The judicial situation- the transplantation law /TPG 6
    Eurotransplant/ET

5. Ethical decision 7
    Living and dying in the comprehension of Christians
    Stance of the Islam

6. Prospering business – trade with organs 8

7. Conclusion.. 9

8. The Sources..10

1. General – What is organ donation?

The life-saving organ transplant can be allowed to seriously ill patients by a post mortal organ donation, so the transference of functioning organs and tissue of a dead to an another person. [1]

An organ donation is the basic condition for a transplant. Condition of the organ donation is the approval of the donator while still alive that in case of a death organs may be taken.

Today by transplantations it's possible to save the life of the patients with organ failure or in improving quality of life decisively. [2]

The aim of such an operation is to restore the function of own organs from the sick people with the help of the taken organs from other people.

The following organs can be successfully transplanted: kidneys, liver, lungs, heart, pancreas and intestines. Hands and faces were added to the transplantation list in 2014. [3]

Not only organs but also tissue can be donated. Referring to the tissues, they let transplant themselves including the skin, the hard skin from the eyes, the heart valves and parts of the blood vessels and the cartilage-tissue.

The body tissue is applicable due to its diversity for the treatment of different injuries, as for example a serious incineration.

Generally the post mortal tissue donations are not transplanted directly after the withdrawal, but are cleaned and preserved in special tissue banks.

For particular organs, such as the kidney or a part of the liver, a living donation is considered under certain circumstances. Nevertheless, the postmortal organ donation has priority before the living donation. [4]

<u>The living donation</u>
The most donations take place as soon as the donor dies, but some organs and tissues can be donated from living donators.[5] In Germany you can only donate a kidney or part of the liver, other organs are not allowed to donate while the donor is alive. Tissue donations are possible, too, for example the transfer of cartilages or bone marrow.

The living donation is subordinated to the post mortal donation: That means, a withdrawal of organs or tissues are only allowed if no post mortal donated organ is available.

---

[1] BZgA: Lebendorganspende – Voraussetzungen und Rahmenbedingungen
[2] https://medlineplus.gov/organdonation.html
[3] https://www.organdonor.gov/about/what.html
[4] https://www.organspende-info.de/kurz-knapp
[5] https://organdonor.gov/about/process/living-donation.html

According to the laws in Germany, the living donation is only allowed between personally connected people. This law should prevent the trade with the organs, and ensure that the living donation is exclusively an act of welfare and charity between two related parties. [6]

There are some requirements you have to fulfil as a living donor:

- Living donors should be physically fit and in good health.
- They have to be of age, most suitably between 18 and 60 years.
- The donation has to be effected voluntarily and without any financial compensation.
- The donors have to be informed about all risks of a living donation and they have to agree to the donation.[7]

2. Process of organ donation – a race against death

For donor organs and tissue, two separate doctors must declare the brain death. The brain death is a surely sign of death, because the essential bodily functions (for example the breathing) are missing without a working brain. That means the person is irretrievably dead.

After this process, the organ procurement coordinator will examine if the dead patient is a registered organ or tissue donor, for example with an organ donor card. [8] If there isn't a written statement, the doctors have to speak with the relatives. These relatives decide about his presumed willingness of the dead patient.

As soon as the brain death is declared and there is an agreement about the donation, the doctors can start with the removal of the suitable organs. This comprises some tests to exclude any dangerous infections and the determination of the blood values. All values will be conveyed to ,,Eurotransplant". The next step is the search of the optimal receiver. And not until then this receiver will be informed that they found a suitable organ.

Immediate after the removal the countdown starts, because the time to transport the taken organs is limited. By way of example, the lungs and the heart have to be obtained and transplanted within five hours. [9]

The organs will be brought to the transplantation centres as fast as can be organized. The receiver is already prepared for the operation, with the result that the operation can begin with the arrival of the donated organ.

After the removal of the organ or the tissue, the corpse will be released for the funeral. In this way, the relatives can take farewell of the departed. [10]

In general, the aftercare for the receiver continues the whole life, because the own organism recognizes the new organ as a foreign object and tries to reject this organ. Therefore regular examinations are imperative. [11]

---

[6] BZgA: Lebendorganspende – Voraussetzungen und Rahmenbedingungen
[7] https://organdonor.gov/about/process/living-donation.html
[8] http://www.cdtny.org/get-informed/the-process/
[9] BZgA: Organspende macht Schule, 2013, Seite 43
[10] http://www.vitanet.de/organspende/ablauf

Figure 1

This depiction shows the whole organ donation process.

For copyright reasons deleted.

Source: http://www.dso.de/fileadmin/templates/media/Uploads/Bilder/Kreisablauf_OS/K01-0-FB-133-0_Kreisdiagramm_Organspende_engl.jpg

This picture depicts the different organs and tissues who can be donated.

3. The situation of organ donations in Germany

The willingness to donate own organs is very high in Germany. About 75% of the German population approved of a removal of organs, but only about 25% possess a written statement.[12]

More than 12.000 patients hope for a suitable organ to save their lives. One single organ donation can enable them to live a new life.[13]

The figure of postmortal organ donations has decreased lately. While in 2010 more than 1.200 people donated their organs after their deaths, in 2014 there were only 846 organ donors in Germany. With this fact, Germany ranks in the last third, compared with other countries in the world.[14]

The waitlist in Germany
For all organs applies: The need of donated organs considerably exceeds the amount of actually donated organs.

Waiting for an organ transplant three people die a day in Germany waiting for an organ transplant because there couldn't be found a suitable organ. That's less than 1000 dead people per year.[15] About a third of the waitlist dies before a suitable organ was found.

Because there are less organs than needed, it's necessary to distribute the ones that are available in a fair way. This way is legally defined and refers to the pressure and the chances for success.[16]

The waiting time for a transplant is in average four to five years. „But the sad truth is that this wait for a suitable organ is often longer than the time you have left."[17]

---

[11] https://www.organspende-info.de/organ-und-gewebespende/verlauf-einer-organ-gewebespende
[12] BZgA: Organspende macht Schule, 2013, Seite 25
[13] BZgA: Organspende macht Schule, 2013, Seite 17
[14] http://www.dso.de/
[15] http://www.dw.com/en/three-die-a-day-in-germany-waiting-for-an-organ-transplant/a-15135297
[16] BZgA: Antworten auf wichtige Fragen, 2012, Warum gibt es lange Wartelisten?

Therefore an organ donation is essential for the people on the waiting list: 100 organ donors more per year, can help about 300 patients to a new life![18]

Figure 2

For copyright reasons deleted.

Source: http://www.dso.de/

This diagram displays the organ donation in Germany from 2010 to 2015.

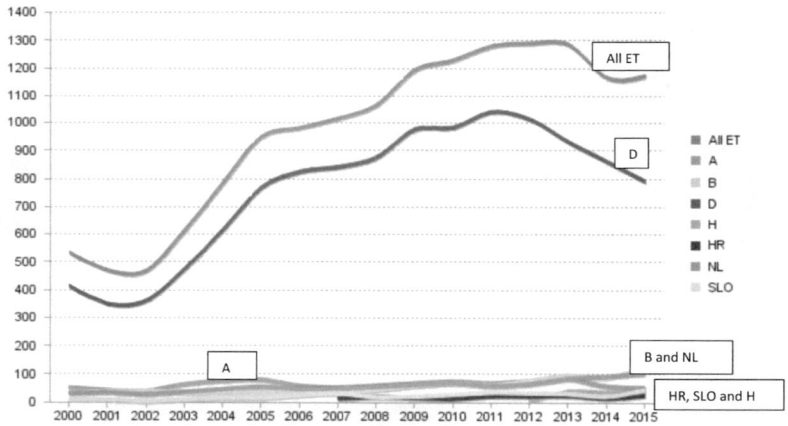

Figure 3

This chart refers to the patients who wait for the different organs in Germany over the course of the years since 2000.

---

[17] http://www.dw.com/en/three-die-a-day-in-germany-waiting-for-an-organ-transplant/a-15135297
[18] Wormer, Eberhard: Lebensrettende Transplantation Organspende, Helmut Lingen Verlag, 2010, Seite 78

4. The judicial situations- the transplantation law /TPG

The transplantation law controls the donation, the removal and the transfer of the organs. Besides, the trade with organs is forbidden in this law.

The TPG created a safe judicial cornerstone, to make the organ donation as transparent as possible. And it tries to exclude every kind of abuse. [19]

The transplantation law includes without limitation this important core points:

- Agreement to the organ or tissue donation

Those who give an explanation for a removal of organs can choose between three options: agree to the donation, disagree or pass the decision to a person you trust. The explanation can be limited to some organs or tissues. The explanation can be given from the 16th birthday. Young persons can also disagree to the organ donation from their 14th birthday too.[20]

- Declaration of death

Organs and tissues only may obtained after the death of the donor is definitely diagnosed. Two independent doctors have to determine the death and to document their conclusion in a written form. [21]

- Transplantation centres and hospitals

Transplantations of organs, for example of the heart, the kidney or the lungs, are allowed in special transplantation centres only. Moreover, the parts of removal, of intervention and of transplantation have to be separated from each other. [22]

- The living donation of organs

A living donation is allowed only when no postmortal donated organ is available. This form of donation is possible between relatives or person close to each other.

- Prohibition of the trade with organs and tissues

It isn't allowed to trade or try to trade with tissues and organs. This offence is sentenced with a prison term up to five years. [23]

Eurotransplant/ET
The transplantation law tries to prevent an abuse of the distribution of the organs. Therefore, it prescribes a central agency, who distributes the organs.

The independent foundation Eurotransplant was founded in 1967, based on the initiative of Johannes J. van Rood.

---

[19] BZgA: Organspende macht Schule, 2013, Seite 25
[20] BZgA: Organspende macht Schule, 2013, Seite 26
[21] http://www.drze.de/in-focus/organ-transplantation/legal-aspects
[22] BZgA: Antworten auf wichtige Fragen, 2012, Was sagt das Transplantationsgesetz?
[23] BZgA: Organspende macht Schule, 2013, Seite 27

Eight nations are members of this association called Eurotransplant. Its members are Germany, Austria, the Netherlands, Belgium, Luxembourg, Croatia, Hungary and also Slovenia. The chance to find a suitable organ rise with this association, because the area has about 120 million inhabitants.

Eurotransplant takes over the key role in the search of a suitable organ and the distribution of these organs. [24] The central assignments of Eurotransplant are: a fair distribution of the organs based on objective medical criterions. [25]

The data of all patients, who wait for a donation of an organ that shall save their life, and the data of the donated organs converge in Eurotransplant. In the very moment the DSO (Deutsche Stiftung Organtransplantation) reports a donor, Eurotransplant determines with computerized support a suitable receiver from the waitlist.

Eurotransplant works over national borders for the common aim of the life-saving transplantation.[26]

5. The ethical decision

The question about the organ donation after death raises not only medical and legal aspects but especially ethical aspects.
Medical progress created good requirements to help people with the organ transplantation. But without the agreement of the people to donate their organs, a transplantation isn't possible. Although the motives are helpfulness and charity it isn't easy to make a decision, because this resolve raises lots of ethical and religious questions. These questions lead to doubt and reflection of the own decision.

Are people allowed to engage in the process of life and death? The human being as a spare parts depot? And there are lots of other questions about the ethical aspects.

The discussion about these questions raises different attitudes. There is no general answer for all people. Everyone has to balance the different aspects for himself, to build his individual opinion. [27]

Living and dying in the comprehension of Christians
The Christians think that the organ donation after the own death is a symbol of solidarity to the ill people. Besides, it is a symbol of helpfulness and charity. In the explanation of the Christian church organ donation is included without limitation: Our life and our body is a present from our God, we can't command about. But we can take advantage of it because of our love to each other.
Those who decide that they want to donate an organ act ethically and religiously, because in this way they can help other people, and give them a ,,second" life. [28]

---

[24] Wormer, Eberhard: Lebensrettende Transplantation Organspende, Helmut Lingen Verlag, 2010, Seite 52
[25] BZgA: Organspende macht Schule, 2013, Seite 45
[26] Wormer, Eberhard: Lebensrettende Transplantation Organspende, Helmut Lingen Verlag, 2010, Seite 52
[27] BZgA: Organspende macht Schule, 2013, Seite 62
[28] BZgA: Antworten auf wichtige Fragen, 2012, Wie stehen die Kirchen zur Organspende?

This attitude may not be enforced. That means if anyone decides against an organ donation, this attitude may not be held against him. [29]

Stance of the Islam

In the Holy Writ, the Koran, there is written, that those who keep one human being alive, do the same as to keeping all people alive.
An organ donation is a good deed after death. The removal and the transplantation are being legally supported. But the transfer of organs may only function for the purpose of charity and definitely not for trade. The Islam people appeal to the population to consider the organ donation and to make the best decision for themselves.[30]

6. Prospering business – trade with organs

Human Organ Trafficking is the trade with human organs for the purpose of illegal organ transplantations.

The demand for donated organs for an organ transplantation is very high due to the many waiting patients. At the end of 2013 about 15.000 people were standing on the waiting list of „Eurotransplant". The legal way isn't enough to compensate this waiting list. This is the reason why some organ dealers provide the organs in illegal ways, especially kidneys and livers.

There are 10.00 - 20.000 illegal transplantations of kidneys per year. That's about 10% of all organ transplantations. [31]

The trade with organs is regulated by the transplantations law in Germany. Nevertheless lots of German patients let transplant themselves illegally acquired organs. Those who wait for a new kidney have to wait about seven years to get a suitable organ. This waiting time is really a great psychological and physical strain for these people. In the course of time more and more bodily functions don't operate anymore. In their special situation applies no-holds-barred for the patients to get a second chance.

If it's a matter of life and death lots of people forget their ethical and moral principles.

While we acquired mainly resources from the economically disadvantaged until now, today people of the developing countries sell their kidneys to us. This involuntary organ donation exists especially in Africa, Brazil, India and Romania. Those who give their organs often suffer from poverty and despair.

Those who sell their organs to the organ dealers hope, that they can live a better life with more safety with the profit gained by the organs. For a donated kidney the vendors receive about 10.000 Euro.

The organ dealers earn at least ten times as much as the donor fee. This proves how lucrative this deal really is for them. The organ dealers have got the biggest advantage of this situation,

---

[29] http://www.dober.de/ethik-organspende/
[30] http://islam.de/files/pdf/organspende
[31] http://www.organhandel.info/organverkauf/

because the body of the donor and the body of the receiver must deal with the problems after the transplantation. [32]

Figure 4

For copyright reasons deleted.

Source: http://bigthink.com/philip-perry/what-you-need-to-know-about-human-organ-trafficking

This picture shows some men who sell their organs to earn money for a better life.

Figure 5

For copyright reasons deleted.

Source: http://bigthink.com/philip-perry/what-you-need-to-know-about-human-organ-trafficking

In this picture the different profits of the organs are depicted.

7. Conclusion – answer to the central question

In summary, it can be stated that lots of things have been pushed forward to give many people a second chance for life in the past years. Nevertheless, the figure of the organ donors decreases very strongly in Germany. That's the reason why lots of people lost their lives, based on the missing donated organ.

To the central question, if a decision for a donation makes sense, I can clearly reply with a YES. Not only the possibility for the receiver, who gets the organ in order to be able to lead a new life, but also the imagination of a survival after death is important to the donor.

The organ donation is a delicate topic: on one side we want to help other people after our death, but on the other side we are afraid of abuse. In general it isn't difficult to save other people's life and to improve the situation of organ donation in Germany.

So I hope more people will inform themselves about the organ donation and at the end more people should document their decision about organ donation in a written form.

---

[32] http://bigthink.com/philip-perry/what-you-need-to-know-about-human-organ-trafficking

8. The sources

Electronical sources

- http://bigthink.com/philip-perry/what-you-need-to-know-about-human-organ-trafficking
- http://islam.de/files/pdf/organspende
- https://medlineplus.gov/organdonation.html
- https://organdonor.gov/about/process/living-donation.html
- https://www.organdonor.gov/about/what.html
- https://www.organspende-info.de/kurz-knapp
- http://www.cdtny.org/get-informed/the-process/
- http://www.dso.de/
- http://www.dw.com/en/three-die-a-day-in-germany-waiting-for-an-organ-transplant/a-15135297
- http://www.drze.de/in-focus/organ-transplantation/legal-aspects
- http://www.dober.de/ethik-organspende/
- http://www.organhandel.info/organverkauf/
- http://www.vitanet.de/organspende/ablauf

Sources of illustrations
Figure 1, Figure 2
- http://www.dso.de/fileadmin/templates/media/Uploads/Bilder/Kreisablauf_OS/K01-0-FB-133-0_Kreisdiagramm_Organspende_engl.jpg

Figure 3
- http://statistics.eurotransplant.org/index.php?search_type=waiting+list&search_region=Germany&search_period=by+year+chart

Figure 4, Figure5
- http://bigthink.com/philip-perry/what-you-need-to-know-about-human-organ-trafficking

- http://www.dermaorgan.gov.my/wp-content/uploads/2013/07/organ.jpg
- https://s-media-cache-ak0.pinimg.com/564x/58/a8/ee/58a8ee27ef32cfda34279a6d3136329b.jpg
- https://s-media-cache-ak0.pinimg.com/originals/66/2e/81/662e8150cb51f90d2e4fed22428dd5b1.jpg
- http://www.hkk.de/uploads/pics/organspende_ablauf.png
- http://www.transplantation-verstehen.de/dotAsset/27055.jpg

Sources of books and magazines

- BZgA: Antworten auf wichtige Fragen, 2012
- BZgA: Lebendorganspende – Voraussetzungen und Rahmenbedingungen
- BZgA: Organspende macht Schule, 2013
- Wormer, Eberhard: Lebensrettende Transplantation Organspende, Helmut Lingen Verlag, 2010

YOUR KNOWLEDGE HAS VALUE

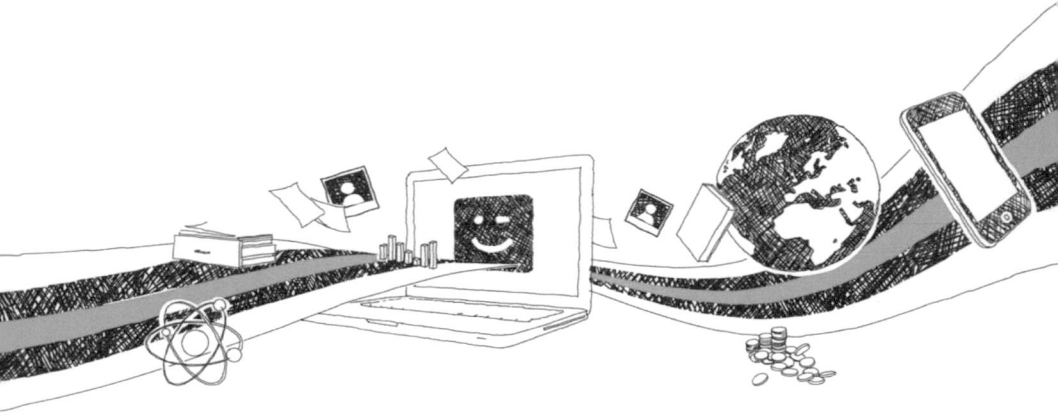

- We will publish your bachelor's and master's thesis, essays and papers

- Your own eBook and book - sold worldwide in all relevant shops

- Earn money with each sale

Upload your text at www.GRIN.com and publish for free

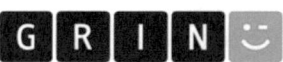